Living with a Narcissist:

Coping Strategies for Emotional Wellness

1. Introduction

2. Understanding Narcissism

3. Recognizing the Signs

4. Psychological and Emotional Impact

5. Coping Mechanisms

6. Survival Strategies

7. Healing and Recovery

8. Moving Forward

9. Conclusion

1. INTRODUCTION

Living with a narcissist can be psychologically demanding and emotionally wearing. Whether it's a friend, relative, boyfriend, or coworker, running into someone with narcissistic symptoms or a full-fledged narcissistic personality disorder (NPD) can seriously affect one's general well-being and mental health. This book seeks to explore the subtleties of narcissism, provide understanding of how it affects relationships, and offer doable coping mechanisms for anyone negotiating this challenging terrain.

Defining Narcissism and Narcissistic Personality Disorder (NPD)

Fundamentally, narcissism is marked by a persistent need for adulation, a lack of empathy for others, and a recurring pattern of grandiosity—in fantasy or conduct. Those with narcissistic personality disorder (NPD) usually show an exaggerated feeling of self-importance, a fixation with fantasies of endless prosperity, power, intelligence, beauty, or perfect love, and a belief they are exceptional and unique. They frequently have a sense of entitlement, demand too much respect, and use people to further their own interests.

Living with a narcissist requires negotiating a complicated web of actions including emotional abuse, gaslighting, manipulation, and a continual demand for validation. For those close to them, these qualities can create a demanding and occasionally poisonous environment that causes great emotional upheaval.

Effects on Mental Health and Well-being of Living with a Narcissist

Living with a narcissist can have rather significant and varied consequences. Among the most often occurring effects are ones on the person's self-worth and self-esteem. Over time, constant criticism, invalidation of emotions, and manipulative strategies can damage one's confidence. The demand for control and adulation of the narcissist can lead to impotence and a loss of autonomy for the other person.

Moreover, in severe circumstances the emotional rollercoaster of being in a relationship with a narcissist can cause anxiety, sadness, and even post-traumatic stress disorder (PTSD). Their erratic emotions and actions might make one feel as though they are constantly attempting to forecast and avoid any confrontations or criticism, therefore walking on eggshells.

Social contacts outside the narcissistic dynamic might also suffer since the person may grow apart from friends and relatives who might not grasp or accept the degree of the narcissist's actions. This solitude might aggravate emotions of hopelessness and loneliness even more.

This book's main objective is to provide direction and doable coping mechanisms for those in relationships with narcissists. It seeks to enable readers with understanding of narcissism, its expressions, and how it affects relationships. Understanding the mechanisms at work helps readers to start recovering their sense of self and investigate approaches for emotional wellness.

The central argument is that although one cannot change a narcissist, one can alter their own reactions and actions to lessen the bad consequences of the relationship. Setting limits, taking care of oneself, and creating coping strategies that advance emotional resilience and well-being all help to foster this.

Narcissistic Behaviors and Patterns

Recognizing and understanding typical actions and patterns linked with NPD is essential for one to properly deal with living with a narcissistic. These might include:

Seeking continuous praise and reinforcement from others, the narcissist often overstates their successes and skills.

Often discounting or denying emotions that do not fit their own, they struggle to relate to the experiences and viewpoints of others.

Narcissists may gaslight individuals and events to keep control or to avoid owning their actions. Gaslighting—which may be quite confusing and destructive—is causing someone to doubt their reality, memory, or perspective.

Sense of Entitlement: They might take advantage of others to meet their own demands or wants without regard to their feelings or welfare.

Narcissists generally have turbulent relationships marked by idealizing (first seeing someone as wonderful or outstanding), devaluation (after degrading or criticizing them), and discard (quickly abandoning relationships when they no longer fit their demands).

Strategies for Emotional Wellness

Living with a narcissist calls for proactive plans and fortitude to preserve psychological and emotional well-being. Although every scenario is different, some generally applicable coping mechanisms include in:

Clearly define the acceptable and inappropriate actions in your life. Tell these limits gently and forcefully; be ready to impose penalties should those limits be broken.

Give self-care activities that advance relaxation, stress reduction, and emotional healing a priority. This could call for yoga, mindfulness meditation, journaling, or joyful and fulfilling hobby pursuits.

Create a support system of reliable friends, relatives, or a therapist able to offer emotional support, affirmation, and perspective. Speaking with others who know your situation can be quite comforting and affirming.

Learning and using assertive communication strategies will help you to properly express your needs, ideas, and emotions without turning to passivity or aggression. Assertiveness advances good relationships and helps to preserve limits.

Educating Yourself: Through reliable sources, books, and articles, boost your knowledge of narcissism and NPD. Understanding helps you to spot manipulative strategies and guide your judgments on contacts and relationships.

Remind yourself that the actions and behaviors of the narcissist have nothing to do with your value or worth personally. Practice self-compassion and challenge bad self-talk resulting from their critiques or invalidations.

Investigating Exit Strategies: Sometimes disengaging or separating oneself from the narcissistic relationship would be the greatest way for emotional well-being. This could entail looking at alternate living quarters, organizing a safe evacuation plan, or consulting legal counsel on divorce or custody issues.

2. Understanding Narcissism

Understanding narcissism means exploring the complex features of narcissistic personality disorder (NPD), the several forms of narcissists, how narcissism develops, and it's significant influence on relationships. Let's go into great detail on every one of these facets:

Features of Narcissistic Personality Disorder (NPD)

Beginning in early life and present in a variety of contexts, Narcissistic Personality Disorder (NPD) is defined by the Diagnostic and Statistical Manual of Mental Disorders (DSM-5) as a pervasive pattern of grandiosity (in fantasy or behavior), a constant need for admiration, and a lack of empathy. Among important traits are:

1. Grandiosity: Believing they are better than others, a narcissist will typically overstate their talents and accomplishments. They are deeply ingrained in need of recognition as distinct and special.

2. Admiration Need: Narcissists' ego is fed by too much appreciation from others. If their expectations are not satisfied, they could grow bitter or dismissive and search for reinforcement and praise.

3. Lack of Empathy: A great lack of empathy is among NPD's most identifying characteristics. Narcissists find it difficult to relate to or concern about the emotions and viewpoints of other people. Often seeing people as less than or useless, they ignore their feelings and wants.

Narcissists have an exaggerated feeling of entitlement, thinking they should be given exclusive treatment and rights. They might use others to satisfy their own needs free from guilt or regret.

Often using manipulative strategies like gaslighting—distorting facts or reality to make someone doubt their own perspective—and exploitation—manipulative behavior helps narcissists preserve their self-image and control over others.

6. Shallow Relationships: Though first charming and charismatic, narcissists usually have shallow and transactional relationships. To get respect and approval, they might idealize others; however, when

those people no longer meet their needs, they devalue and reject them.

Kinds of Narcissists and Their Behavior Styles

Different manifestations of narcissism result in numerous acknowledged kinds or subtypes:

1. Grandiose narcissist: This kind shows overt conceit, self-importance, and an insatiable demand for appreciation. Often seeking high-status roles, they may show off their wealth or accomplishments conspicuously.

2. Vulnerable Narcissist: Often referred to as covert narcissists, they seem modest or meek but really suffer from extreme sensitivity to criticism and inadequacy. By acting passively-aggressive or with self-pity, they could control others.

3. Malignant Narcissist: This subtype blends antisocial behavior, violence, lack of regret, and narcissistic qualities with antisolic tendencies. To

keep their sense of control, they could show sadistic tendencies or love hurting others.

4. Communal Narcissist: On the surface, these people seem unselfish and charitable; nonetheless, they demand appreciation for their alleged giving. They may utilize deeds of compassion to control people and improve their self-esteem.

5. Somatic Narcissist: Somatic narcissists give their physical appearance, health, or sexual ability much attention. They may exploit their beauty to control others and search for continual approval and appreciation of their physical features.

How Narcissism Emerges and Affects Relationships

Complex and affected by a confluence of genetic, environmental, and psychological elements is the development of narcissism:

1. Early Life Events: Early events such extreme pampering or neglect, uneven parental attention, or unreasonable praise and expectations can all lead to narcissism. These encounters could cause a fragile self-esteem and a need for outside approval to grow.

2. Personality Attributes: Some personality traits, such perfectionism, a strong need for power or control, or a lack of empathy, could make people prone to grow narcissistic tendencies.

3. Environmental Conditions: Emphasizing success, competitiveness, and individuality in society could help to support narcissistic behavior. Cultural standards that give success and status top priority help to foster narcissistic qualities.

4. Impact on Relationships: Narcissism seriously strains relationships and frequently results in emotional conflict and dysfunction:

5. Devaluation and Idealization: Originally idealizing their spouses, narcissists often set them on a pedestal

and pay them lots of respect and attention. But this idealization is often fleeting, replaced by devaluation when the spouse questions the narcissist's ego or falls short of demanding standards.

6. Control and Manipulation: To keep control over their spouses, narcissists employ gaslighting, guilt-tripping, or emotional blackmail—manageable strategies. They could make their partner emotionally reliant by taking advantage of weaknesses and fears.

7. Emotional abuse: Emotional abuse can follow from a lack of empathy and contempt of others' emotions. Narcissists undermine their partners' self-esteem by belittling, criticizing, or demeaning them, therefore generating a poisonous dynamic.

8. Cycles of Idealization, Devaluation, and Discard: Relationships with narcissists frequently follow a set pattern of idealizing, devaluing, and discarding. The spouse could feel confused, hurt, and emotionally worn out as well as strong highs and lows.

For those impacted by narcissistic relationships, understanding these characteristics is absolutely essential. It helps spouses or family members create plans to safeguard their own well-being and negotiate the difficulties of living with or relating to someone with narcissistic personality disorder.

It also offers understanding of why narcissists behave the way they do. The first step in putting good coping mechanisms into use and encouraging emotional wellness in these challenging situations is realizing the indicators and actions of narcissism.

3. Recognizing the Signs

Seeing the Symptoms of Narcissism

Relationships can be seriously affected by narcissism, a personality feature marked by grandiosity, a continuous desire for praise, and a lack of empathy. Maintaining emotional well-being and creating reasonable limits depend on early identification of narcissistic qualities in a friend, relative, or spouse. This article investigates typical actions displayed by narcissists, red flags that act as early warning signals, and techniques for spotting these qualities in different kinds of relationships.

Approaching Narcissistic Features

Clinically, Narcissistic Personality Disorder (NPD) is a diagnostic for a spectrum of behaviors distinguished by an exaggerated sense of self-importance, a profound need for too much attention and admiration, disrupted relationships, and a lack of empathy for others. Although not everyone displaying narcissistic qualities has NPD, knowing these symptoms will assist one negotiate difficult interpersonal relationships.

Typical Behaviors Showed by Narcissists

One of the traits of narcissists is grandiosity and exaggeration of their accomplishments, skills, or value. Their exaggerated feeling of self-importance makes them prone to continual validation and adulation from others.

Usually absent in narcissists is empathy—that is, the capacity to understand and share another person's feelings. Focusing mostly on their own needs and wants, they could discount or minimize the emotions and hardships of others.

1. Sense of Entitlement: Narcissists sometimes have irrational expectations of good treatment. Without

necessarily proving suitable behavior or effort, people could feel they merit particular advantages or accolades.

Narcissists can be rather manipulative in order to keep their inflated self-image and power over others. To reach their objectives, they could turn to flattery, guilt, or dishonesty, therefore subverting the autonomy of others.

2. Difficulty Handling Criticism: Narcissists may view even small setbacks or criticism as personal attacks, which may cause defensiveness, rage, or withdrawing behavior. They could respond disproportionately to supposed slights or challenges to their authority.

3. Preoccupation with Status and Appearance: Narcissists give their image and status first priority. As a form of respect and validation, they could be unduly fixated on worldly goods, social standing, or physical looks.

For narcissists, accepting responsibility for their acts or owning their mistakes can be difficult. To get out from under penalties, they could rationalize their behavior, assign guilt to others, or create excuses.

Early Warning Signs and Red Lights

Early recognition of narcissistic features helps people preserve their emotional well-being and make wise judgments concerning their relationships. Typical red flags include:

For narcissists seeking control and respect, love bombing — intense first attention and affection followed by a rapid progression into a relationship—can be a strategy.

Dominating talks about oneself, undervaluing of others' contributions, and disinterest in others' life indicate narcissistic behavior.

Common among narcissists is a disregard of personal boundaries, like invading personal space, obtaining private information without permission, or making decisions without consulting others.

A hallmark of narcissistic behavior is emotional manipulation — using guilt, fear, or obligation to drive others into compliance or to meet their needs.

Frequently used by narcissists is gaslighting — managing someone into doubting their own reality, memory, or sanity in order to keep control and undercut their confidence.

Characteristic of narcissistic behavior are shallow shows of empathy or sympathy that do not follow into real actions or support.

Extreme charm and violence, generosity and selfishness, or devotion and contempt can all point to unstable narcissistic tendencies when alternated.

Acknowledging Narcissistic Elements in Various Relationships

Especially in the framework of close relationships, family dynamics, or friendships, recognizing narcissistic behaviors can be difficult. In romantic relationships, first appeal and charm can soon give place to emotional manipulation and control. To prevent setting off their partner's fears or fury, partners may find themselves always treading on eggshells.

In family settings, narcissistic features might show themselves in a parent who puts their personal wants before their children's emotional well-being, therefore depriving their children of nurturing or affirmation. Extended family members or siblings could also show narcissistic traits, therefore generating negative dynamics inside the family.

Among friends, narcissistic qualities could show up as envy, rivalry, or a relentless demand for approval and affirmation. Friends could feel used or controlled by someone who only appreciates their output or perspective on the narcissist's image.

Coping and Boundary Strategies

Once one recognizes narcissistic qualities, one must give self-care top priority and set limits to safeguard mental health:

Knowing narcissistic features and behaviors will allow you to confirm your experiences and define what is and isn't appropriate behavior in relationships.

Clearly state your boundaries and expectations of how you wish to be handled. Should limits be regularly violated, be ready to enforce penalties.

Talk to reliable friends, relatives, or a therapist who can offer viewpoint, affirmation, and direction on negotiating relationships with narcissistic people.

Give your own emotional well-being a priority; practice self-compassion; participate in joyful and fulfilling activities.

Seeking professional counseling or therapy might offer coping mechanisms and recovery from the consequences of narcissistic relationships in circumstances of extreme manipulation or emotional abuse.

Final Thought:

Maintaining good relationships and safeguarding one's emotional well-being depend on one realizing narcissistic qualities in a friend, relative, or boyfriend. Understanding common behaviors displayed by narcissists, spotting red flags and early warning indications, and putting coping mechanisms and limited limits into use will help people negotiate difficult interpersonal dynamics with more awareness and resilience. In the end, giving self-care top priority and looking for help will help to create loving, respectful, and mutually happy relationships.

4. Psychological and Emotional Impact

Emotional and psychological effects of living with a narcissist

Living with a narcissist can have severe psychological and emotional effects on one's general mental health, self-esteem, and self-worth. The effects of narcissistic behavior on individuals, the emotional manipulation strategies usually utilized by narcissists, and the destructive behaviors such as gaslighting and blame-shifting that aggravate these effects are investigated in this essay.

Affects Self-Esteem and Self-Worth

Constant demand for affirmation and adulation by narcissists sometimes comes at the expense of others' self-esteem and self-worth. Living with a narcissist might cause an individual to experience the following:

To keep their own sense of superiority, narcissists could disparage, devalue, or ignore the accomplishments and skills of others. This might undermine the person's confidence and sense of ability over time.

Narcissists give their own needs and wants top priority above others, therefore neglecting, undervaluing, or underlining persons in the connection.

Constant gaslighting and manipulation can cause people to doubt their own impressions, memories, and judgment. This self-doubt permeates

all facets of their lives and fuels indecision and
anxiety.

People who try to satisfy the narcissist and
avoid conflict may start looking for outside validation
and acceptance instead of depending on their own gut
sense and emotions.

Narcissists could cut off people from their
support system by dictating who they can spend time
with, disparaging their connections, or staging drama
that drives others off. This solitude might aggravate
loneliness and reliance on the narcissist even more.

Living with a narcissist sometimes entails
cycles of idealizing (love bombing), devaluation
(criticism and manipulation), and discard (ignoring
or abandonment of the individual). Emotionally
taxing and disruptive these cycles can be.

Emotional Strategies Narcissists Employ

Different strategies are used by narcissists to dominate and influence others, therefore supporting their sense of power and superiority:

Gaslighting is a psychological manipulation strategy used by narcissists to make you doubt your sanity, memory, or judgment by either negating or distorting facts, events, or your perspective of reality. They might refuse to admit, for instance, that they spoke nasty words or blame you of seeing unrealistically occurring difficulties.

When faced with their conduct or mistakes, narcissists frequently point the finger elsewhere. They could deny their own accountability, embellish the flaws of others, or shift the focus to make themselves the victim.

Narcissists project onto others their own bad qualities, emotions, or behaviors. Should they be unfaithful, for example, they might accuse their partner of adultery. This projection helps to shift focus from their own actions and assign guilt elsewhere.

Particularly at social events or when they desire something from others, narcissists can be quite seductive and appealing. This appeal might cover their deceptive inclinations and make it challenging for others to see their detrimental actions.

Common among narcissists is emotional blackmail — using guilt, fear, or responsibility to compel people into meeting their expectations. Unless their wants are satisfied, they could threaten to deny affection, encouragement, or resources.

In relationships, narcissists may establish triangles by incorporating a third party (such as harshly discussing someone behind their back) to generate separation and take control over the dynamics between people.

Gaslighting, Blame-Shifting, and Other Harmful Behaviors

Key components of narcissistic manipulation strategies and can have terrible consequences on individuals are gaslighting, blame-shifting, and other destructive behaviors:

Gaslighting compromises the personal reality and sense of events perception. It generates uncertainty, self-doubt, and a loss of confidence in one's own judgment, therefore generating anxiety, despair, and emotional instability.

Deflecting blame on others helps narcissists avoid owning their behavior and control others into feeling guilty or responsible for issues in the relationship. Shame, inadequacy, and frustration can all follow from this.

The instability of a narcissistic relationship—alternating between strong love and affection (idealization) and criticism or disinterest (devaluation)—creates an emotional rollercoaster for the individual. Increased worry, hyper-vigilance, and emotional tiredness can all follow from this instability.

Constant criticism, insults, and insulting comments from a narcissist amount to emotional violence. This gradually reduces the person's self-esteem, feeling of value, and emotional fortitude.

Narcissists ignore the effects on others as they shape reality to fit their demands and wants. This manipulation can skew the person's view of what is appropriate or healthy in relationships, therefore sustaining cycles of emotional upheaval and instability.

To keep power and dominance in the relationship, narcissists may cut off people from their support network, control their finances or decisions, and prescribe conduct. Feelings of loneliness, dependability, and helplessness can all follow from this solitude.

Managing Stress and Getting Help

Healing and restoring personal well-being starts with realizing the psychological and emotional toll living with a narcissist causes:

Honor the manipulation and abuse you have gone through to legitimize your emotions and start to reconstruct your sense of self.

Clearly define your boundaries with the narcissist to safeguard your emotional well-being and implement penalties should those boundaries be crossed.

Speak with close friends, relatives, or a therapist who can offer affirmation, viewpoint, and direction on negotiating narcissistic relationships.

Give activities and practices that advance your mental, emotional, and physical well-being—such as exercise, hobbies, meditation, or time spent with encouraging people top priority.

Discover narcissistic personality traits and manipulative strategies to help you to better grasp the dynamics at work and empower yourself with knowledge.

Professional counseling or therapy can offer techniques for healing from emotional abuse, rebuilding self-esteem, and changing interpersonal habits.

Final Thought:

Living with a narcissist can have very negative psychological and emotional effects on general well-being, self-esteem, and self-worth. Understanding the manipulation strategies used by narcissists—such as gaslighting and blame-shifting—helps one to better identify and lessen their influence. To negotiate these difficult relationships and promote personal healing and development, one must first give self-care top priority, set limits, get help, and learn about narcissistic behaviors. Key first stages toward recovering a better and more fulfilled life free from the impact of narcissistic abuse are ultimately recovering autonomy and developing resilience.

5. Coping Mechanisms

Coping Mechanisms for Managing Narcissistic Relationships

Living or engaging with a narcissist can be emotionally taxing. Coping mechanisms are critical tools for preserving your mental and emotional health while navigating these difficult interactions. This essay investigates successful coping tactics, such as setting boundaries, building a support network, practicing self-care through mindfulness and therapy, and improving assertiveness and communication skills.

Establishing and Maintaining Boundaries

When interacting with a narcissist, it is critical to set clear boundaries to protect your emotional health and feeling of autonomy. Here is how to successfully set and enforce boundaries:

1. Identify Your Limits: Consider what behaviors and interactions are acceptable or unacceptable to you. This clarity will lead you in establishing limits that are consistent with your values and requirements.

2. Communicate Clearly: Communicate your boundaries to the narcissist in a calm and strong tone. Use "I" statements to describe how their actions affect you and what you require to feel respected and protected.

3. Consistency is Key: Narcissists may test or push limits in order to keep control. It's critical to continually establish your boundaries and resist manipulation or guilt-tripping tactics.

4. Prepare for Resistance: Expect the narcissist to resist or test your boundaries. Maintain your resolve and remind yourself that prioritizing your own well-being is not selfish, but rather vital for strong relationships.

5. Seek Support: Discuss your limits with trusted friends, family, or a therapist who can offer support and validation. They can also provide perspective and keep you accountable to your boundaries.

Building a Support Network

Building a support network is critical for emotional affirmation, guidance, and practical assistance while dealing with narcissistic relationships:

1. Identify Supportive Individuals: Surround yourself with people who understand and validate your feelings. These people can provide empathy, wisdom, and a sense of camaraderie.

2. Diversify Your Support: Seek help from a variety of sources, including friends, family, support groups, and online forums. Each source can offer unique viewpoints and ways of support.

3. Set Boundaries with Supportive Others: Communicate your requirements and boundaries to your support network so that they may provide constructive help without adding unnecessary stress or pressure.

4. Professional Support: Consult a therapist or counselor who specializes in narcissistic abuse. They can provide suggestions for coping, healing, and building healthier relationship habits.

5. Join Support Groups: Meeting with others who have faced similar issues can provide validation,

understanding, and techniques for dealing with narcissistic behavior.

Self-Care Strategies: Mindfulness, Therapy, and Stress Management.

Self-care is critical for sustaining resilience and mitigating the stress associated with narcissistic relationships:

1. Mindfulness and Meditation: Practice mindfulness techniques, such as meditation or deep breathing exercises, to increase present-moment awareness and minimize worry and rumination.

2. Therapy and Counseling: Therapy can provide a safe environment to process feelings, gain insight into interpersonal dynamics, and create coping techniques tailored to your individual circumstance.

3. Healthy Lifestyle Choices: Put physical health first by eating nutritious foods, exercising regularly, and

getting enough sleep. Physical well-being has a substantial impact on emotional resiliency.

4. Creative Outlets: Find creative activities or hobbies that make you happy and allow you to express yourself freely. This can be a good way to relieve stress and emotional tension.

5. Reserve Relaxation Time: Plan regular breaks or relaxation sessions to unwind and recharge. This could involve reading, bathing, spending time in nature, or engaging in a pastime.

Assertiveness Training and Communication Skills

Developing assertiveness and communication skills will help you manage interactions with narcissists more effectively.

1. Assertiveness Techniques: Use assertive communication to convey your opinions, feelings, and needs directly and politely. Maintain eye contact and project confidence.

2. Develop Clear Expectations: Clearly convey your expectations for the narcissist's behavior and interactions. Be clear about what you require to feel respected and appreciated in the relationship.

3. Active Listening: Actively and empathetically listen to the narcissist's problems or points of view while remaining mindful of your own needs and boundaries. Recognize their viewpoint while asserting your own.

4. Avoid JADE (Justify, Argue, Defend, Explain): Narcissists might start disputes or manipulate conversations. Avoid excessive self-justification or explanation. Stick to your boundaries and priorities.

5. Develop Patience and Persistence: Assertiveness might be difficult at first, particularly in emotionally charged settings. Practice tolerance with yourself and keep using aggressive communication strategies.

Final Thought:

Coping with narcissistic relationships involves deliberate effort and a number of tactics for safeguarding your emotional well-being and establishing healthy boundaries. Individuals can navigate these difficult dynamics with greater resilience and confidence by establishing and consistently enforcing clear boundaries, building a strong support network, prioritizing self-care through mindfulness and therapy, and improving assertiveness and communication skills.

It's crucial to remember that obtaining professional help and practicing self-compassion are critical components of properly dealing with narcissistic behavior. Finally, prioritizing your own well-being and cultivating healthy connections are critical steps toward regaining autonomy and emotional stability in the midst of narcissistic issues.

6. Survival Strategies

Strategies for Survival in Living with a Narcissist

Being around a narcissist can be emotionally draining. Using survival techniques will enable people to keep their sanity, emotional balance, and general well-being in daily contacts. This article offers doable advice on how to negotiate life with a narcissist, keep emotional balance, and create reasonable expectations to properly handle setbacks.

Useful Advice for Daily Living Among Narcissists

Living daily with a narcissist calls for calculated strategies to reduce conflict and preserve emotional stability:

Not every problem has to be faced; Choose Your Battles - Choose which problems you should resolve and which you may let go to keep your mental clarity.

Limit emotional participation in the actions of the narcissist by means of Practicing Emotional Detachment. Rather of trying to shape or control theirs, concentrate on your own reactions and feelings.

Set Clear Boundaries: Tell the narcissist firmly and establish, for yourself, clear boundaries. Regularly enforce these limits to safeguard your health.

Try to avoid trigger topics—that is, those that usually cause conflict or manipulation—by means of avoidance whenever at all possible.

Talk to the narcissist short, factual, and with an eye toward pragmatic concerns. Reduce sharing of sensitive information or weaknesses that might be turned against you.

Create a support system of reliable friends, relatives, or a therapist who can offer emotional support, affirmation, and direction at trying circumstances.

Practice Self-Care: Give exercises, hobbies, meditation, or time in nature top priority for activities that support emotional resilience, stress release, and leisure.

Keeping a notebook or diary of your interactions with the narcissist will help you to validate your experiences and obtain understanding of behavioral patterns.

How to Save Your Sanity and Emotional Balance

Living with a narcissist calls for deliberate self-care and coping mechanisms to help you to stay sane and emotionally balanced:

Even if the narcissist seeks to discount or ignore your feelings, Valuate Your Feelings and accept them. Trust your impressions; then, ask for confirmation from encouraging others.

Using meditation, deep breathing exercises, or grounding techniques, develop mindfulness to remain present and lower anxiety or rumination.

Spend time in settings where you feel comfortable and supported to help you to minimize your contact to the manipulative actions of the narcissist.

Invest time and effort in pursuits that support your own development, pleasure, and fulfillment free from the narcissist's validation or approval.

Set Realistic Expectations: Understand that the behavior or personality of the narcissist is not changeable. Change your expectations to help to lower disappointment and irritation.

Avoid self-blame since the actions of the narcissist is not your responsibility. Avoid absorbing their judgment or linking their behavior to your own failings.

To help you process your feelings, get perspective on the dynamics of the relationship, and create coping mechanisms fit for your situation, think about therapy or counseling.

Maintaining empathy and respect for yourself and others, assertively express your needs and limitations.

Control Disappointments and Create Realistic Expectations

Maintaining your emotional health and negotiating the difficulties of living with a narcissist depend on your having reasonable expectations:

One should be aware that the narcissist might not modify their behavior or give your requirements first priority. Pay attention to your controllable factors, such limits and reactions.

Outside of your relationship with the narcissist, clear priorities and principles. To keep a feeling of direction and contentment, spend time and effort in activities that fit these priorities.

The narcissist might not live up to your standards for empathy, validation, or support, so be ready for disappointments. Create resilience plans that help you to move on from disappointment.

Validate your own achievements, feelings, and value free from the narcissist's approval. Positive affirmations and self-care help to build self-esteem.

Manage Emotional factors: Determine in your contacts with the narcissist factors that cause disappointment or irritation. Plan ways to control these triggers and keep emotional equilibrium.

See from reliable friends, relatives, or a therapist who can provide ideas and encouragement in handling setbacks and negotiating relationship difficulties.

Even in the middle of challenging conditions with the narcissist, **celebrate tiny victories** and times of personal development.

Final Thought

Living with a narcissist calls for resilience, self-awareness, and pragmatic techniques as well as emotional balance preservation. Practical advice for daily contacts, self-care and emotional stability, reasonable expectations, and effective management of disappointment can help people negotiate the complexity of narcissistic relationships with more resilience and autonomy.

Recall that managing and prospering in demanding interpersonal dynamics depend critically on practicing self-compassion and asking for help from reliable others. In the end, emphasizing your own well-being and personal development will help you to negotiate narcissistic relationships with more clarity, strength, and emotional health.

7. Healing and Recovery

Healing and Recovery From Narcissistic Relationships

Recovering from narcissistic relationships may be a difficult road with emotional scars and a feeling of lost self-worth. Essential first stages toward reclaiming your life and promoting personal development are realizing you need professional treatment, looking at therapy choices including individual counseling and support groups, and emphasizing rebuilding confidence. This article explores these facets in order to offer direction on the road towards recovery from narcissistic abuse.

Understanding When One Should See a Professional

Those in recovery from narcissistic relationships must learn when to seek professional treatment. These indicators point to possible professional support being helpful:

If your daily life is disrupted by continuous sadness, worry, rage, or thoughts of worthlessness, you are persistent emotional distress.

If you find it difficult to manage unwanted ideas, memories, or emotional triggers connected to prior events with the narcissist,

If you feel isolated from others, steer clear of social events or battle mistrust of people resulting from prior emotional abuse.

Engaging in activities such drug abuse, self-harm, or dangerous activity as a means of emotional healing is self-destructive behavior.

Effect on Relationships: Should residual emotional scars sour your contacts with friends, relatives, or colleagues?

If you feel cut off from your sense of self, interests, or passions that were eclipsed during the connection with the narcissist, you are **losing**.

If you find yourself caught in habits of action or thinking that reinforce guilt, humiliation, or inadequacy,

Therapy Choices: Support Groups, Individual Counseling

Therapy offers a safe and encouraging setting where one may grow coping mechanisms, get understanding of interpersonal dynamics, and process emotions. Common therapeutic choices for recovering from narcissistic relationships include:

Individual counseling—that is, private exploration of your ideas, feelings, and experiences under the direction of a certified therapist or counselor—allows you to Therapists can assist you in developing better coping strategies, healing from emotional scars, and seeing behavior trends.

Emphasizing the identification and modification of negative thinking patterns and actions causing emotional discomfort, Cognitive Behavioral Therapy (CBT), enables people to grow in more flexible approaches of thinking and handling demanding circumstances.

Trauma-informed therapy is helpful for people who have gone through emotional or psychological trauma—including that of narcissistic abuse. Therapists assist clients process trauma, lower symptoms of post-traumatic stress, and rebuild trust and safety using specific approaches.

Joining a support group for people who have suffered narcissistic abuse offers shared experiences, validation, and peer support. Support groups can create a feeling of connection, help to lower loneliness, and offer doable healing and recovery guidance.

Eye Movement Desensitization and Reprocessing (EMD) is a therapy technique used in

EMDR Therapy to assist people process traumatic events and lessen their emotional impact. Focusing on upsetting memories or triggers, it entails directed eye motions or other types of bilateral stimulation.

Focus of psychodynamic therapy is on investigating unconscious ideas and patterns of behavior resulting from past relationships or childhood events. It enables people to understand fundamental problems causing present emotional conflicts.

Mindfulness-Based Therapies (MBSR) or mindfulness-based cognitive therapy (MBCT) can help people build present-moment awareness, lower anxiety, and improve emotional control abilities.

Rebuilding Your Life and Confidence

Recovering self-confidence and taking back your life from narcissistic abuse calls both self-compassion and deliberate work. These techniques help to promote personal development and empowerment:

Spend some time reestablishing your values, interests, and strengths—that which could have been eclipsed in the marriage. Investigate joyful and fulfilling new pastimes or past interests.

Replace self-criticism with self-affirming words and to Challenge Negative Self-Talk. Learn to identify and question negative self-perceptions the narcissist may have reinforced.

Break down more ambitious objectives into smaller, doable actions. No matter how little they seem, celebrate your advancement and achievements all along.

Learn to assertively express in relationships your wants, values, and boundaries. Surround yourself with encouraging people that value your limits.

Prioritize activities that support physical, emotional, and mental well-being—exercise, healthy diet, enough sleep, and relaxation techniques—by means of which you practice self-care.

Let go of shame or self-blame for keeping in the relationship or suffering mistreatment. Acknowledge that given the tools and knowledge at the time, you performed the best you could.

As you heal and develop, nurture supportive relationships with friends, relatives, or members of a support group that offer validation, empathy, and encouragement.

If at all feasible, use journaling, letter writing—even if you don't send it—or closure activities advised by your therapist to assist process unresolved feelings and events.

Final Thought:

Recovering from narcissistic relationships requires realizing you need professional treatment, investigating therapy choices including support groups and individual counseling, and emphasizing developing self-confidence and reclaiming your life.

Those who seek help from experienced therapists, join supportive communities, and practice self-care and self-compassion will be more resilient and empowered as they negotiate the healing path. Recall that healing is a slow process needing patience, introspection, and a dedication to give your own well-being top priority. Over time and effort, you can come out of narcissistic abuse stronger, more self-aware, and ready to welcome a better, fulfilled life.

8. Moving Forward

Moving Forward: Creating a Contented Life Beyond Relationships Based on Narcissism

Reclaiming personal pleasure, development, and stability requires first moving ahead from a narcissistic relationship. This essay looks at ways to assess your choices—that of staying or divorcing the relationship—as well as useful advice for co-parenting with a narcissist (if relevant) and creating a happy life free from the impact of narcissistic dynamics.

Examining Your Alternatives: Choosing to Leave or Stay in a Relationship

Making the difficult and personal choice to stay in or leave a narcissistic relationship calls for serious thought of several elements:

1. Evaluating Safety: Give your emotional and physical safety top priority. Should you or your kids

be at danger for abuse or harm, divorcing the partnership could be required to ensure your safety.

2. Think about how the connection influences your general happiness, self-esteem, and mental wellness. Think about whether keeping in the relationship affects your well-being or adds to continuous emotional pain.

3. See a therapist or counselor knowledgeable in narcissistic abuse for professional direction. They can help you investigate choices for going forward, confirm your experiences, and offer objective observations.

4. Investigating Change and Growth: Determine whether the narcissist is ready to use therapy or another intervention to recognize and modify their conduct. Change in narcissistic personality features, however, might be difficult and unrealistic at times.

5. If you choose to break off the relationship, assess your financial condition and if you have the resources to sustain yourself and any dependents.

6. Think about the availability of emotional, pragmatic, and financial help during the change from friends, family, or support groups.

7. Long-Term Goals: Match your choices to your values, long-term plans for your family and yourself. Determine whether keeping in the relationship fits your idea of personal development and fulfillment.

Techniques for Co-Parenting with a Narcissist

Because of their domineering demeanor, lack of empathy, and quest of power and dominance, co-parenting with a narcissist might offer special difficulties. These techniques help you negotiate co-parenting so as to minimize conflict and give your children's welfare top priority:

Define and explain to the narcissistic co-parent exact limits on communication, decision-making, and parenting obligations. Always stay inside these limits.

Pay mostly attention to the children since their best interests should be first. Decisions should be focused on what is physically and emotionally healthy for the child, not on following power battles with the narcissistic parent.

Consider parallel parenting if direct contact with the narcissistic parent is difficult or explosive. This entails, where needed, minimizing physical contact and communicating via written means or outside third-party mediators.

Record any correspondence you send to the narcissistic co-parent, including emails, messages, and notes from in-person meetings. Legal uses as well as custody conflicts can benefit from this material.

See a family law attorney with background in high-conflict custody issues for legal advise. They can offer direction on your legal rights, choices for deciding on custody, and techniques for safeguarding the welfare of your children.

Help your kids to recognize appropriate limits and coping mechanisms for handling the conduct of the narcissistic parent. Promote honest communication and validate their emotions without discounting the other parent's.

Practice Self-Care: Give self-care top priority so you might be emotionally free from the actions of the narcissistic parent. Take breaks; ask for help from close friends or therapists; and participate in leisure activities meant to help with stress and relaxation.

Constructing a Content Life Outside of the Narcissistic Relationship

Constructing a happy life apart from a narcissistic relationship is a path of self-discovery, healing, and personal development. These techniques help you to develop resilience and recover your sense of happiness and identity:

Invest time and effort in rediscovering your hobbies, passions, and values—that which the marriage could have overlooked. Participate in things you enjoy and find fulfilling.

Create reasonable objectives for personal development, professional advancement, or academic interests. To create momentum and acknowledge your development, break out more ambitious projects into doable steps.

Surround yourself with loving friends, relatives, or a community that validate your experiences, offer encouragement, and raise your spirits through trying circumstances.

Accept chances for education, personal growth, or new experiences that will broaden your horizons and provide new angles on life outside the boundaries of the narcissistic relationship.

Release emotions of resentment, rage, or bitterness toward the narcissistic ex-partner by means of practice for forgiveness and let-off. Embrace an attitude of acceptance and self-compassion and work on forgiving yourself for any alleged inadequacies.

Establish a daily schedule that gives self-care—including enough sleep, healthy food, frequent exercise, and mindfulness techniques that support emotional well-being top priority.

Over the healing process, identify and honor your talents, resiliency, and personal development. Honor your development and confirmations of your value and ability.

Final Thought:
From a narcissistic relationship, moving on calls for clear, self-awareness-based evaluation of your options, careful handling of co-parenting issues (if

any), and active building of a satisfying life free from the impact of narcissistic dynamics.

Individuals can start a road of healing, resilience, and reclaiming their sense of identity and fulfillment by giving their safety, well-being, and long-term goals top priority; by seeking help from reliable professionals and supportive networks; by embracing chances for personal development and happiness; Healing is a trip that plays out at its own speed; each step forward you are recovering your power and helping to shape a better future for yourself and the people you love.

9. Conclusion

Final Thought: Authorizing Yourself in Narcissistic Relationships

From identifying symptoms and behaviors to coping mechanisms, healing techniques, pushing advancing with resilience, we have explored many components during our examination of narcissistic relationships. This last chapter seeks to summarize important ideas and techniques covered, offer support for giving well-being top priority, and empower people negotiating relationships with narcissists.

Review of Important Points and Approaches Addressed

1. Recognizing Signs and Behaviors: We have found typical narcissist qualities like grandiosity, lack of empathy, manipulation, and a continuous need for adulation. Knowing these qualities helps one negotiate relationships and create reasonable limits.

2. Important coping strategies are setting limits, building a support system, using mindfulness and therapy to practice self-care, and improving assertiveness and communication abilities. These techniques help people to negotiate the difficulties presented by narcissistic relationships and safeguard their emotional well-being.

3. Important first steps in healing from narcissistic abuse are realizing you need professional help, looking at therapy choices including individual counseling and support groups, and emphasizing developing self-confidence. Healing is confirming one's experiences, organizing emotions, and recovering a feeling of autonomy and identity.

4. Examining choices for either staying or leaving a relationship requires weighing safety, emotional impact, and long-term goals. Approaches for co-parenting a narcissist stress establishing limits, putting children's welfare first, and, where needed, consulting attorneys. Reconnecting with oneself,

establishing personal goals, developing supportive relationships, and seizing fresh chances for development and satisfaction help one to build a satisfying life outside of narcissistic dynamics.

Inspired to Give Well-Being Top Priority

In negotiating relationships with narcissists, you must give your well-being top priority. Here is the rationale:

One value is your mental and emotional wellbeing. Setting limits, giving self-care top priority, and getting help are not selfish behaviors—rather, they are required for your general wellbeing.

Acknowledging and knowing narcissistic characteristics helps you to empower yourself to make wise judgments on how to react and guard yourself from emotional damage or control.

From therapy seeking to self-compassion practice, every action performed toward healing and recovery increases resilience and develops your capacity to overcome obstacles and flourish.

Giving your health top priority can help others —including children or loved ones impacted by the narcissistic dynamics—to set a strong example. It shows fortitude, dignity, and the bravery to follow a better route.

Hope and Empowerment for Those Dealing with a Narcissist

Although living with or interacting with a narcissist can feel isolated and taxing, you have hope and empowerment right at your disposal:

1. Many people have followed a similar road and found means of navigating and recovering from narcissistic relationships. Ask for help from close friends, relatives, or support groups who can be sympathetic and motivating based on your experiences.

2. Your Voice Matters: Your needs, feelings, and experiences are real. Though the narcissist tries to discredit or devaluate your instincts and observations, trust them.

3. Embracing Change: Although the behavior of the narcissist might be unusual, you have the ability to start good changes in your own life. Pay attention to your controllable actions—your choices, reactions, and personal development.

4. Celebrate every step forward, no matter how little. Every limit you establish, every moment of self-care, every choice you make in your best interest is a victory deserving of recognition.

5. You deserve pleasure, fulfillment, and a life free of emotional manipulation or abuse. Accept chances for development, follow your interests, and surround yourself with encouraging people.

Final Thought:

Negotiating narcissistic relationships calls for bravery, fortitude, and a dedication to give your health top priority. Individuals can recover their sense of identity and create happy lives outside of narcissistic dynamics by identifying indications and behaviors, utilizing successful coping techniques, getting professional help when needed, and emphasizing healing and personal development.

Remember; your path is different and healing happens at its own speed. Accept every advance with hope for the future and empathy for yourself. You are strong and resilient enough to flourish outside of narcissistic relationships and design a life full of authenticity, happiness, and empowerment.